Blood Type O Meal Plan and Food List

A Custom Eating Plan and Blood Type O Food, Beverage and Supplement Lists

Rosalee Casper

Copyright © 2024 by Rosalee Casper

Table of Contents

Introduction

Understanding Blood Type O: An Overview

Blood type O is one of the four main blood types, alongside A, B, and AB, determined by the presence or absence of certain antigens on the surface of red blood cells. Understanding the characteristics and implications of blood type O is crucial for tailoring dietary choices and lifestyle habits to optimize health and well-being.

Blood type O is characterized by the absence of A and B antigens on red blood cells, leaving only the O antigen present. This genetic makeup is inherited from one's parents, with specific combinations of genes determining an individual's blood type.

Research suggests that blood type O may have evolved among early humans, particularly those with hunter-gatherer lifestyles. Individuals with blood type O are theorized to have adapted to diets rich in animal proteins and low in grains and dairy, reflecting the dietary patterns of ancient hunter-gatherer societies.

Individuals with blood type O often exhibit certain physiological characteristics that may influence health and dietary needs. These traits include robust immune systems, efficient metabolism, and a tendency toward higher levels of stomach acid production.

Blood type O is believed to influence how the body responds to different foods, with proponents of the blood type diet theory suggesting that individuals with blood type O may benefit from a diet rich in lean proteins, fruits, and vegetables while limiting grains, dairy, and legumes. This dietary approach aims to optimize digestion, energy levels, and overall health based on blood type-specific considerations.

While the blood type diet theory remains a topic of debate among scientists and nutrition experts, there is growing recognition of the importance of personalized nutrition approaches. Understanding one's blood type, including blood type O, can provide valuable insights into potential dietary sensitivities, nutrient needs, and overall health considerations.

How Blood Type O Affects Diet and Nutrition

Understanding how blood type O influences diet and nutrition is essential for individuals seeking to optimize their health and well-being through personalized dietary choices. From digestion to nutrient metabolism, various factors contribute to the unique dietary needs of individuals with blood type O.

Digestive Efficiency and Protein Metabolism:

Individuals with blood type O are often characterized by robust digestive systems, particularly in their ability to metabolize and digest animal proteins efficiently. This trait is believed to stem from ancestral dietary patterns that prioritized animal-based foods, such as meat and fish. As a result, blood type O individuals may thrive on diets rich in lean meats, poultry, and fish, which provide essential amino acids necessary for muscle growth, repair, and overall health.

Carbohydrate Tolerance and Grain Sensitivity:

Contrary to other blood types, individuals with blood type O may exhibit lower tolerance to certain carbohydrates, especially those derived from grains and legumes. This is attributed to the historical avoidance of agricultural products in ancestral diets, favoring a hunter-gatherer lifestyle. As such, blood type O individuals may benefit from minimizing their intake of grains, particularly wheat and corn, and instead focusing on carbohydrate sources from fruits, vegetables, and select grains like rice and quinoa.

Lectin Sensitivity and Food Reactivity:

Lectins are proteins found in various foods that may interact with blood type-specific antigens, potentially triggering immune responses or disrupting metabolic processes. Some proponents of the blood type diet theory suggest that individuals with blood type O may be more sensitive to certain lectins found in grains, legumes, and dairy products. Consequently, limiting or avoiding these foods may help mitigate potential adverse reactions and support optimal health in blood type O individuals.

Optimizing Nutrient Intake and Dietary Balance:

While there are general dietary recommendations for blood type O individuals, personalized nutrition remains key to meeting individual nutrient needs and achieving dietary balance. Emphasizing nutrient-dense foods such as lean proteins, fruits, and vegetables while minimizing processed foods, sugars, and artificial additives can support overall health and vitality. Additionally, incorporating regular physical activity and adequate hydration further complements a blood type O-friendly lifestyle.

Adapting to Individual Variability and Preferences:

It's important to recognize that dietary needs and preferences can vary widely among individuals, even within the same blood type category. Factors such as age, gender, activity level, and underlying health conditions can influence dietary requirements and preferences. Therefore, adopting a flexible approach to dietary planning and experimentation can help individuals with blood type O identify optimal dietary patterns that align with their unique needs and goals.

Chapter 1: Blood Type O Foods to Embrace

1.1 High-Quality Proteins for Blood Type O

Proteins play a crucial role in the diet of individuals with blood type O, providing essential amino acids necessary for muscle growth, repair, and overall health. Selecting high-quality protein sources that align with the unique metabolic tendencies and dietary preferences of blood type O individuals is key to supporting optimal health and vitality.

1. Lean Animal Proteins:

Blood type O individuals thrive on diets rich in lean animal proteins, reflecting their ancestral connection to hunter-gatherer societies. Sources of lean animal proteins include:

- Poultry: Chicken, turkey, and duck are excellent sources of lean protein for blood type O individuals. Opt for skinless cuts and avoid heavily processed or breaded options.

- Beef: Lean cuts of beef such as sirloin, tenderloin, and flank steak provide ample protein without excessive fat content. Grass-fed and organic options are preferred when available.

- Lamb: Lean cuts of lamb, such as loin chops or leg meat, offer a flavorful protein option for blood type O individuals. Trim visible fat to reduce saturated fat intake.

- Game Meat: Wild game meats such as venison, bison, and elk are nutrient-dense protein sources that align with the dietary preferences of blood type O individuals. These meats are typically lower in fat and higher in protein compared to conventionally raised meats.

2. Fish and Seafood:

Fish and seafood are integral components of the blood type O diet, providing valuable protein, omega-3 fatty acids, and essential nutrients. Opt for wild-caught and sustainably sourced varieties whenever possible. Suitable options include:

- Salmon: Rich in omega-3 fatty acids and protein, wild-caught salmon is an excellent choice for blood type O individuals. Avoid farm-raised salmon, which may contain higher levels of contaminants.

- Tuna: Albacore tuna, yellowfin tuna, and skipjack tuna are nutritious protein sources for blood type O individuals. Choose canned tuna packed in water or olive oil to minimize added fats and sodium.

- Sardines: Sardines are a nutrient-dense protein source packed with omega-3 fatty acids, calcium, and vitamin D. Enjoy them fresh, canned in water, or lightly smoked for a flavorful addition to meals.

- Shellfish: Shrimp, crab, lobster, and mussels are protein-rich options that offer variety and versatility in the blood type O diet. Choose fresh or frozen shellfish over breaded or heavily processed varieties.

3. Plant-Based Protein Options:

While animal proteins are emphasized in the blood type O diet, plant-based protein sources can also complement meals and provide additional nutritional benefits. Suitable plant-based protein options include:

- Legumes: Some legumes, such as lentils and black-eyed peas, may be consumed in moderation by blood type O individuals. Soaking and sprouting legumes can help reduce lectin content and improve digestibility.

- Nuts and Seeds: Almonds, walnuts, pumpkin seeds, and chia seeds are nutrient-dense protein sources that can be incorporated into the blood type O diet. Enjoy them as snacks, toppings, or additions to salads and smoothies.

- Soy Products: Non-GMO fermented soy products such as tempeh and miso may be consumed occasionally by blood type O individuals. However, soybeans and soy-based products should be limited due to their lectin content and potential impact on hormone balance.

1.2 Beneficial Fruits and Vegetables

Incorporating a variety of fruits and vegetables into the diet is essential for individuals with blood type O to ensure optimal nutrient intake, support digestion, and promote overall health and well-being. Certain fruits and vegetables are particularly beneficial for blood type O individuals due to their compatibility with their metabolic tendencies and potential health-promoting properties.

1. Dark Leafy Greens:

Dark leafy greens such as spinach, kale, Swiss chard, and collard greens are nutrient powerhouses rich in vitamins, minerals, and phytonutrients. These vegetables are excellent sources of iron, calcium, vitamin K, and antioxidants, supporting bone health, cardiovascular function, and immune health in blood type O individuals.

2. Cruciferous Vegetables:

Cruciferous vegetables like broccoli, cauliflower, Brussels sprouts, and cabbage offer numerous health benefits for blood type O individuals. These vegetables are rich in fiber, vitamins, and antioxidants, promoting digestive health, detoxification, and immune function. Additionally, cruciferous vegetables contain compounds that may support hormone balance and reduce the risk of certain cancers.

3. Berries:

Berries such as blueberries, strawberries, raspberries, and blackberries are nutritional powerhouses packed with antioxidants, vitamins, and fiber. These fruits provide blood type O individuals with a delicious and nutritious way to support immune function, cognitive health, and cardiovascular health. Enjoy berries as a snack, mixed into yogurt or oatmeal, or blended into smoothies for a burst of flavor and nutrition.

4. Citrus Fruits:

Citrus fruits like oranges, grapefruits, lemons, and limes are rich in vitamin C, antioxidants, and fiber, making them valuable additions to the blood type O diet. These fruits support immune health, collagen production, and cardiovascular function, while also enhancing the flavor and freshness of dishes. Incorporate citrus fruits into salads, marinades, and beverages for a tangy and refreshing twist.

5. Root Vegetables:

Root vegetables such as sweet potatoes, carrots, beets, and parsnips offer blood type O individuals a nutritious source of carbohydrates, vitamins, and minerals. These vegetables provide sustained energy, support blood sugar regulation, and contribute to digestive health and satiety. Roast, steam, or mash root vegetables as side dishes or incorporate them into soups, stews, and casseroles for added flavor and nutrition.

6. Apples and Pears:

Apples and pears are versatile fruits that provide blood type O individuals with a satisfying combination of fiber, vitamins, and antioxidants. These fruits support digestive health, blood sugar regulation, and cardiovascular function, while also offering a naturally sweet and refreshing taste. Enjoy apples and pears as snacks, sliced onto salads, or baked into healthy desserts for a nutritious treat.

1.3 Incorporating Healthy Fats

Including healthy fats in the diet is essential for individuals with blood type O to support various bodily functions, including hormone production, brain health, and nutrient absorption. Choosing the right types of fats and incorporating them into meals can promote overall health and well-being for blood type O individuals.

1. Omega-3 Fatty Acids:

Omega-3 fatty acids are essential fats that play a crucial role in heart health, brain function, and inflammation regulation. Blood type O individuals can benefit from including sources of omega-3 fats in their diet, such as:

- Fatty Fish: Wild-caught salmon, mackerel, sardines, and trout are excellent sources of omega-3 fatty acids. Incorporating these fish into meals two to three times per week can provide blood type O individuals with a significant amount of these beneficial fats.

- Flaxseeds and Chia Seeds: Ground flaxseeds and chia seeds are plant-based sources of alpha-linolenic acid (ALA), a type of omega-3 fatty acid. Blood type O individuals can sprinkle these seeds on salads, yogurt, or oatmeal to boost their omega-3 intake.

- Walnuts: Walnuts are another plant-based source of omega-3 fatty acids, offering blood type O individuals a convenient and nutritious

snack option. Adding walnuts to salads, smoothies, or baked goods can increase omega-3 consumption while providing satisfying crunch and flavor.

2. Monounsaturated Fats:

Monounsaturated fats are heart-healthy fats that can help lower LDL (bad) cholesterol levels and reduce the risk of heart disease. Blood type O individuals can incorporate sources of monounsaturated fats into their diet, including:

- Avocados: Avocados are rich in monounsaturated fats, fiber, and various vitamins and minerals. Blood type O individuals can enjoy avocados sliced onto toast, mashed into guacamole, or added to salads for a creamy and nutritious addition.

- Olive Oil: Extra virgin olive oil is a staple in the Mediterranean diet and provides blood type O individuals with a flavorful and versatile cooking oil. Use olive oil for sautéing vegetables, dressing salads, or drizzling over

roasted meats and fish to add healthy fats and enhance flavor.

- Nuts and Seeds: Almonds, cashews, pistachios, and sesame seeds are rich in monounsaturated fats and make convenient and satisfying snack options for blood type O individuals. Enjoy a handful of nuts or seeds as a snack or incorporate them into meals for added crunch and nutrition.

3. Coconut Oil:

Coconut oil is a source of medium-chain triglycerides (MCTs), which are a type of saturated fat that may offer various health benefits, including improved cognitive function and weight management. Blood type O individuals can use coconut oil for cooking, baking, or adding flavor to smoothies and desserts in moderation.

4. Nut Butters:

Natural nut butters made from almonds, peanuts, or cashews can provide blood type O individuals with a delicious and nutritious source of healthy fats.

Spread nut butter on whole grain toast, use it as a dip for fruits or vegetables, or add it to smoothies for a creamy and satisfying texture.

1.4 The Importance of Organic and Non-GMO Choices

Opting for organic and non-GMO (genetically modified organism) foods is paramount for individuals with blood type O to minimize exposure to potentially harmful pesticides, herbicides, and genetically engineered ingredients. Choosing organic and non-GMO options can support overall health, reduce the risk of adverse health effects, and align with the principles of a blood type O-friendly diet.

1. Avoiding Harmful Chemicals:

Organic foods are grown and produced without synthetic pesticides, herbicides, and fertilizers, reducing the risk of exposure to harmful chemicals. Blood type O individuals may be particularly sensitive to certain environmental toxins, making organic choices essential for supporting overall health and well-being.

2. Preserving Nutrient Density:

Organic farming practices prioritize soil health and biodiversity, resulting in crops that are often higher in essential nutrients and antioxidants. Blood type O individuals can benefit from consuming organic fruits, vegetables, and grains that retain their nutrient density and offer superior taste and flavor compared to conventionally grown counterparts.

3. Supporting Environmental Sustainability:

Choosing organic foods supports environmentally sustainable agricultural practices that prioritize soil conservation, water quality, and biodiversity. By opting for organic options, blood type O individuals can contribute to environmental conservation efforts and promote long-term sustainability for future generations.

4. Minimizing Exposure to GMOs:

Genetically modified organisms (GMOs) are organisms whose genetic material has been altered through genetic engineering techniques. While the long-term health effects of GMO consumption are still debated, blood type O individuals may choose to avoid GMOs as a precautionary measure. Opting for non-GMO foods can help minimize exposure to genetically engineered ingredients and potential health risks associated with GMO consumption.

5. Supporting Local and Sustainable Agriculture:

Choosing organic and non-GMO foods often involves supporting local farmers and producers who prioritize sustainable farming practices and environmental stewardship. Blood type O individuals can explore farmers' markets, community-supported agriculture (CSA) programs, and local food cooperatives to access a variety of organic and non-GMO foods while supporting their local economy and agricultural community.

6. Reading Labels and Certifications:

When selecting organic and non-GMO foods, blood type O individuals should familiarize themselves with food labels and certifications to ensure they are making informed choices. Look for labels such as USDA Organic, Non-GMO Project Verified, and Certified Organic to identify products that meet organic and non-GMO standards.

Chapter 2: Foods to Avoid for Blood Type O

2.1 Understanding Avoidance Foods for Blood Type O

Identifying and avoiding specific foods that may not align with the metabolic tendencies and dietary preferences of blood type O individuals is essential for promoting optimal health and well-being. Understanding which foods to avoid can help blood type O individuals minimize digestive discomfort, reduce inflammation, and support overall vitality.

1. Lectin-Rich Foods:

Lectins are proteins found in certain foods that may interact with blood type-specific antigens and potentially cause adverse reactions in sensitive individuals. Blood type O individuals may be particularly sensitive to lectins found in:

- Grains: Wheat, barley, rye, and products containing gluten may contain lectins that can exacerbate digestive issues and inflammation in blood type O individuals. Avoiding or minimizing consumption of these grains can help alleviate symptoms and support digestive health.

- Legumes: Beans, lentils, soybeans, and peanuts are rich in lectins and may cause digestive discomfort and bloating in blood type O individuals. Limiting intake of legumes or opting for properly prepared and soaked varieties can reduce lectin content and improve digestibility.

2. Dairy Products:

Dairy products such as milk, cheese, and yogurt contain lactose, a type of sugar that may be challenging for blood type O individuals to digest due to lower levels of lactase enzyme activity. Additionally, dairy products may contribute to inflammation and mucous production in sensitive individuals. Blood type O individuals may choose to limit or avoid dairy products and explore alternative options such as:

- Plant-Based Milk Alternatives: Almond milk, coconut milk, and oat milk are dairy-free alternatives that offer blood type O individuals a nutritious and easily digestible option for enjoying milk-like beverages.

- Non-Dairy Yogurts: Coconut yogurt, almond yogurt, and soy yogurt are dairy-free alternatives that provide blood type O individuals with probiotics and beneficial bacteria for supporting gut health without the potential digestive issues associated with dairy-based yogurts.

3. Processed and Refined Foods:

Processed and refined foods often contain added sugars, unhealthy fats, and artificial additives that can contribute to inflammation, insulin resistance, and weight gain in blood type O individuals. Avoiding or minimizing consumption of processed and refined foods such as:

- Packaged Snacks: Chips, cookies, candy, and other packaged snacks often contain refined sugars, unhealthy fats, and artificial additives that offer little nutritional value and may negatively impact blood sugar levels and overall health.

- Fast Food and Takeout: Fast food and takeout meals are typically high in unhealthy fats, sodium, and refined carbohydrates, making them an unwise choice for blood type O individuals seeking to optimize their health and well-being. Instead, prioritize home-cooked meals made from whole, unprocessed ingredients.

4. Red Meat and Processed Meats:

While blood type O individuals may thrive on diets rich in lean animal proteins, excessive consumption of red meat and processed meats may increase the risk of cardiovascular disease, cancer, and other health issues. Limiting intake of red meat and processed meats such as:

- Beef: Fatty cuts of beef, processed beef products (e.g., bacon, sausage, hot dogs), and cured meats may contain unhealthy fats, preservatives, and additives that can negatively impact health outcomes in blood type O individuals.

- Pork: Pork products such as bacon, ham, and processed pork sausages should be consumed in moderation due to their high levels of saturated fat, sodium, and nitrates/nitrites, which may increase the risk of chronic diseases.

2.2 Lectins and Their Impact on Blood Type O

Lectins are proteins found in various foods that can interact with blood type-specific antigens, potentially affecting digestion, immune function, and overall health in individuals with blood type O. Understanding the impact of lectins on blood type O individuals is essential for making informed dietary choices and optimizing health outcomes.

1. Lectins and Digestive Health:

Certain lectins, particularly those found in grains, legumes, and dairy products, can bind to the lining of the digestive tract and interfere with nutrient absorption, leading to digestive discomfort, bloating, and inflammation. Blood type O individuals may be particularly sensitive to lectins due to their genetic makeup and metabolic tendencies, making it important to minimize consumption of lectin-rich foods.

2. Lectins and Immune Function:

Lectins have the ability to stimulate the immune system and trigger inflammatory responses in sensitive individuals, potentially contributing to autoimmune conditions, food sensitivities, and chronic inflammation. Blood type O individuals may experience heightened immune reactivity to certain lectins, leading to increased susceptibility to allergies, autoimmune disorders, and other immune-related health issues.

3. Lectins and Blood Type O:

Research suggests that blood type O individuals may be more susceptible to the adverse effects of certain lectins compared to individuals with other blood types. This is attributed to the unique composition of blood type O antigens, which may interact with specific lectins in a way that triggers immune responses or disrupts metabolic processes. As a result, blood type O individuals may benefit from limiting or avoiding lectin-rich foods such as:

- Grains: Wheat, barley, rye, and products containing gluten contain lectins that may exacerbate digestive issues and inflammation in blood type O individuals.
- Legumes: Beans, lentils, soybeans, and peanuts are rich in lectins and may cause digestive discomfort and bloating in blood type O individuals.
- Dairy Products: Dairy products such as milk, cheese, and yogurt contain lectins and lactose that may be challenging for blood type

O individuals to digest, leading to digestive issues and immune reactivity.

4. Strategies for Minimizing Lectin Exposure:

Blood type O individuals can minimize their exposure to lectins and mitigate potential adverse effects by adopting the following dietary strategies:

- Focus on Whole, Unprocessed Foods: Prioritize whole, unprocessed foods such as lean proteins, fruits, vegetables, nuts, and seeds that are naturally low in lectins and rich in nutrients.
- Proper Food Preparation: Soaking, sprouting, fermenting, or cooking lectin-rich foods can help reduce lectin content and improve digestibility for blood type O individuals.
- Individualized Approach: Pay attention to how specific foods affect your digestion, energy levels, and overall well-being, and tailor your diet accordingly to minimize lectin exposure and optimize health outcomes.

2.3 Harmful Foods and Ingredients to Steer Clear Of

Identifying and avoiding harmful foods and ingredients is crucial for individuals with blood type O to support optimal health, prevent digestive discomfort, and minimize the risk of inflammation and other adverse health effects. Understanding which foods to steer clear of can empower blood type O individuals to make informed dietary choices and prioritize foods that align with their metabolic tendencies and nutritional needs.

1. Gluten-Containing Grains:

Grains containing gluten, such as wheat, barley, and rye, contain proteins that may trigger adverse reactions in blood type O individuals, including digestive issues, inflammation, and immune reactivity. Avoiding gluten-containing grains and products made from refined flour can help minimize digestive discomfort and support overall well-being for blood type O individuals.

2. Dairy Products:

Dairy products, including milk, cheese, yogurt, and ice cream, contain lactose, a type of sugar that may be challenging for blood type O individuals to digest due to lower levels of lactase enzyme activity. Additionally, dairy products may contribute to inflammation, mucous production, and immune reactivity in sensitive individuals. Steering clear of dairy products can help alleviate digestive issues and support optimal health for blood type O individuals.

3. Processed and Refined Foods:

Processed and refined foods often contain added sugars, unhealthy fats, and artificial additives that can contribute to inflammation, insulin resistance, and weight gain in blood type O individuals. Avoiding or minimizing consumption of processed and refined foods such as packaged snacks, fast food, sugary beverages, and convenience meals can help maintain stable blood sugar levels, support healthy weight management, and reduce the risk of chronic diseases.

4. Artificial Sweeteners:

Artificial sweeteners such as aspartame, saccharin, and sucralose are commonly found in diet sodas, sugar-free snacks, and low-calorie products marketed to individuals seeking to reduce sugar intake. However, these artificial sweeteners may disrupt gut microbiota, increase cravings for sweet foods, and contribute to metabolic dysfunction in blood type O individuals. Steer clear of artificial sweeteners and opt for natural sweeteners such as stevia, monk fruit, or raw honey in moderation.

5. Trans Fats and Hydrogenated Oils:

Trans fats and hydrogenated oils are artificial fats created through the hydrogenation process and commonly found in margarine, shortening, fried foods, and processed baked goods. These unhealthy fats can increase LDL (bad) cholesterol levels, promote inflammation, and raise the risk of heart disease and other chronic conditions in blood type O individuals. Avoiding foods containing trans fats and hydrogenated oils can support cardiovascular health and overall well-being.

6. High-Sugar Foods and Beverages:

High-sugar foods and beverages, including candy, sugary snacks, sweetened beverages, and desserts, can lead to rapid spikes and crashes in blood sugar levels, contributing to fatigue, cravings, and metabolic imbalances in blood type O individuals. Limiting intake of high-sugar foods and opting for natural, whole food sources of sweetness such as fruits, dates, or raw honey can help stabilize blood sugar levels and support energy levels throughout the day.

Chapter 3: Crafting Your Blood Type O Meal Plan

3.1 Designing a Balanced Meal Plan for Blood Type O

Creating a balanced meal plan tailored to the unique metabolic tendencies and dietary preferences of blood type O individuals is essential for promoting optimal health, supporting energy levels, and maintaining overall well-being. By incorporating a variety of nutrient-dense foods and strategic meal timing, blood type O individuals can optimize their diet to meet their nutritional needs and achieve their health goals.

1. Emphasize Lean Proteins:

Start by prioritizing lean protein sources such as poultry, fish, and lean cuts of beef or lamb. These protein-rich foods provide essential amino acids for muscle growth, repair, and overall health. Aim to include a serving of lean protein with each meal to support satiety and maintain muscle mass.

2. Incorporate Abundant Vegetables:

Load up on non-starchy vegetables such as dark leafy greens, cruciferous vegetables, peppers, tomatoes, and cucumbers. These nutrient-packed veggies provide fiber, vitamins, minerals, and antioxidants while adding volume and flavor to meals. Aim to fill half of your plate with colorful vegetables to support digestive health and promote overall vitality.

3. Include Healthy Fats:

Include sources of healthy fats such as avocados, nuts, seeds, and olive oil in your meal plan. These heart-healthy fats provide essential fatty acids, support brain function, and promote satiety. Add a serving of nuts or seeds to salads, drizzle olive oil over roasted vegetables, or enjoy avocado slices as a topping or side dish.

4. Opt for Complex Carbohydrates:

Choose complex carbohydrates such as sweet potatoes, quinoa, brown rice, and oats to provide sustained energy and support blood sugar regulation. These fiber-rich foods offer a steady release of glucose into the bloodstream, preventing spikes and crashes in blood sugar levels. Incorporate complex carbohydrates into meals to fuel workouts, promote satiety, and support overall health.

5. Balance with Fruits and Berries:

Include a variety of fruits and berries in your meal plan to satisfy your sweet tooth and provide essential vitamins, minerals, and antioxidants. Opt for low-glycemic fruits such as berries, apples, pears, and citrus fruits to minimize blood sugar fluctuations. Enjoy fruit as a snack, dessert, or topping for yogurt or oatmeal to add natural sweetness and nutrition to your meals.

6. Practice Portion Control:

Be mindful of portion sizes and listen to your body's hunger and fullness cues. Aim to eat balanced meals that include a combination of protein, carbohydrates, and fats to promote satiety and prevent overeating. Use smaller plates and bowls to help control portion sizes and avoid mindless snacking.

3.2 Meal Prep Tips and Tricks

Meal preparation is a key component of maintaining a healthy and balanced diet, especially for individuals with blood type O. By investing time in meal prep, you can ensure that nutritious and blood type-appropriate meals are readily available, making it easier to stick to your dietary goals and support your overall well-being. Here are some tips and tricks to streamline your meal prep process:

1. Plan Your Meals:

Start by planning your meals for the week ahead. Consider your schedule, dietary preferences, and nutritional needs when creating your meal plan. Choose recipes that are blood type O-friendly and can be easily prepared in bulk.

2. Make a Grocery List:

Once you have your meal plan in place, create a detailed grocery list to ensure you have all the ingredients you need. Organize your list by food categories to make shopping more efficient and avoid forgetting any essential items.

3. Batch Cook Protein and Grains:

Spend some time batch cooking lean proteins such as chicken, turkey, fish, and lean cuts of beef or lamb. Cook grains such as quinoa, brown rice, or oats in large batches as well. Portion them out into meal-sized containers for easy grab-and-go options throughout the week.

4. Prep Vegetables in Advance:

Wash, chop, and pre-portion your vegetables ahead of time to save time during the week. Store them in airtight containers or zip-top bags to keep them fresh. You can also roast or steam vegetables in advance to have them ready to add to salads, stir-fries, or grain bowls.

5. Utilize Slow Cookers and Instant Pots:

Slow cookers and Instant Pots are excellent tools for batch cooking meals with minimal effort. Use them to prepare soups, stews, chili, or shredded meats that can be portioned out and enjoyed throughout the week.

6. Pre-Pack Snacks and Smoothie Ingredients:

Prepare individual portions of snacks such as nuts, seeds, sliced fruits, or veggie sticks for easy grab-and-go options. You can also pre-pack smoothie ingredients in freezer bags or containers, so all you have to do is blend them with your choice of liquid when you're ready to enjoy a nutritious smoothie.

7. Incorporate Variety:

Don't be afraid to experiment with different recipes and flavors to keep your meals exciting and satisfying. Incorporate a variety of proteins, grains, vegetables, and seasonings to create balanced and flavorful meals.

8. Use Portion-Controlled Containers:

Invest in portion-controlled containers or meal prep containers to help you portion out your meals and prevent overeating. These containers make it easy to pack lunches for work or school and ensure that you're sticking to appropriate portion sizes.

9. Stay Organized and Flexible:

Keep your kitchen organized and stocked with essential ingredients and meal prep tools to streamline the process. Be flexible and willing to adjust your meal plan as needed based on changes in your schedule or preferences.

Chapter 4: Sample Blood Type O Meal Plans

4.1 One-Week Blood Type O Meal Plan

Day 1	
Breakfast	Scrambled eggs with spinach and mushrooms cooked in olive oil.
Snack	Sliced apple with almond butter.
Lunch	Grilled chicken salad with mixed greens, cherry tomatoes, cucumber, and avocado. Dress with olive oil and lemon juice.
Snack	Carrot sticks with hummus.
Dinner	Baked salmon served with quinoa and steamed broccoli.
Day 2	
Breakfast	Greek yogurt topped with mixed berries and a sprinkle of chia seeds.

Snack	Handful of mixed nuts (almonds, walnuts, cashews).
Lunch	Turkey lettuce wraps filled with sliced turkey breast, avocado, bell peppers, and shredded carrots.
Snack	Celery sticks with peanut butter.
Dinner	Stir-fried beef with bell peppers, onions, and broccoli served over brown rice.
Day 3	
Breakfast	Oatmeal cooked with almond milk, topped with sliced banana and a drizzle of honey.
Snack	Cherry tomatoes with mozzarella cheese.
Lunch	Quinoa salad with black beans, corn, diced tomatoes, avocado, and cilantro. Dress with lime juice and olive oil.
Snack	Sliced cucumber with tahini.

Dinner	Grilled shrimp skewers with zucchini and bell peppers served with a side of roasted sweet potatoes.
Day 4	
Breakfast	Smoothie made with spinach, banana, almond milk, and protein powder.
Snack	Handful of trail mix (dried fruit and nuts).
Lunch	Lunch: Lentil soup with carrots, celery, onions, and kale.
Snack	Apple slices with cheese.
Dinner	Baked chicken thighs with roasted Brussels sprouts and quinoa.
Day 5	
Breakfast	Scrambled tofu with sautéed kale and cherry tomatoes.
Snack	Edamame beans.
Lunch	Tuna salad with mixed greens, cucumber, cherry tomatoes, and olives. Dress with olive oil and balsamic vinegar.

Snack	Bell pepper strips with guacamole.
Dinner	Beef stir-fry with broccoli, bell peppers, and snap peas served over cauliflower rice.
Day 6	
Breakfast	Avocado toast on whole grain bread topped with sliced tomatoes and a sprinkle of sea salt.
Snack	Greek yogurt with honey and sliced almonds.
Lunch	Chicken and vegetable soup with barley.
Snack	Baby carrots with hummus.
Dinner	Grilled lamb chops with roasted asparagus and sweet potato wedges.
Day 7	
Breakfast	Smoothie bowl topped with granola, mixed berries, and shredded coconut.
Snack	Hard-boiled eggs.
Lunch	Spinach salad with grilled chicken, strawberries, almonds, and balsamic vinaigrette.

Snack	Sliced pear with cheese.
Dinner	Baked halibut with steamed green beans and quinoa pilaf.

4.2 Two-Week Blood Type O Meal Plan

Day 1	
Breakfast	Scrambled eggs cooked in olive oil with spinach and tomatoes.
Snack	Sliced apple with almond butter.
Lunch	Grilled chicken salad with mixed greens, bell peppers, cucumber, and avocado. Dress with olive oil and lemon juice.
Snack	Carrot sticks with hummus.
Dinner	Baked salmon served with quinoa and steamed broccoli.
Day 2	
Breakfast	Greek yogurt topped with mixed berries and chia seeds.

Snack	Handful of mixed nuts (almonds, walnuts, cashews).
Lunch	Turkey lettuce wraps filled with sliced turkey breast, avocado, bell peppers, and shredded carrots.
Snack	Celery sticks with peanut butter.
Dinner	Stir-fried beef with broccoli, onions, and snap peas served over brown rice.
Day 3	
Breakfast	Oatmeal cooked with almond milk, topped with sliced banana and a drizzle of honey.
Snack	Cherry tomatoes with mozzarella cheese.
Lunch	Quinoa salad with black beans, corn, diced tomatoes, avocado, and cilantro. Dress with lime juice and olive oil.
Snack	Sliced cucumber with tahini.

Dinner	Grilled shrimp skewers with zucchini and bell peppers served with a side of sweet potatoes.
Day 4	
Breakfast	Smoothie made with spinach, banana, almond milk, and protein powder.
Snack	Trail mix (dried fruit and nuts).
Lunch	Lentil soup with carrots, celery, onions, and kale.
Snack	Apple slices with cheese.
Dinner	Baked chicken thighs with roasted Brussels sprouts and wild rice.
Day 5	
Breakfast	Avocado toast on whole grain bread topped with sliced tomatoes and a sprinkle of sea salt.
Snack	Greek yogurt with honey and sliced almonds.
Lunch	Chicken and vegetable stir-fry with broccoli, bell peppers, and snap peas served over cauliflower rice.

Snack	Baby carrots with hummus.
Dinner	Grilled lamb chops with roasted asparagus and quinoa pilaf.

Day 6

Breakfast	Scrambled tofu with sautéed kale and cherry tomatoes.
Snack	Edamame beans.
Lunch	Tuna salad with mixed greens, cucumber, cherry tomatoes, and olives. Dress with olive oil and balsamic vinegar.
Snack	Bell pepper strips with guacamole.
Dinner	Beef stir-fry with broccoli, onions, and snap peas served over cauliflower rice.

Day 7

Breakfast	Smoothie bowl topped with granola, mixed berries, and shredded coconut.
Snack	Hard-boiled eggs.
Lunch	Spinach salad with grilled chicken, strawberries, almonds, and balsamic vinaigrette.

Snack	Sliced pear with cheese.
Dinner	Baked halibut with steamed green beans and quinoa pilaf.
Day 8	
Breakfast	Quinoa porridge topped with sliced bananas and a drizzle of maple syrup.
Snack	Handful of trail mix (mixed nuts and dried fruit).
Lunch	Grilled turkey burgers served on whole grain buns with lettuce, tomato, and avocado.
Snack	Celery sticks with almond butter.
Dinner	Baked cod fillets with roasted vegetables (zucchini, bell peppers, onions) and a side of sweet potato wedges.
Day 9	
Breakfast	Smoothie made with spinach, pineapple, coconut milk, and protein powder.
Snack	Greek yogurt with honey and sliced almonds.

Lunch	Lentil and vegetable curry served with brown rice.
Snack	Carrot and cucumber sticks with hummus.
Dinner	Grilled chicken breast with steamed broccoli and quinoa pilaf.
Day 10	
Breakfast	Scrambled eggs with sautéed spinach and mushrooms.
Snack	Apple slices with peanut butter.
Lunch	Tuna salad stuffed in a whole grain pita pocket with lettuce and tomato.
Snack	Mixed berries with cottage cheese.
Dinner	Beef stir-fry with bell peppers, snap peas, and broccoli served over cauliflower rice.
Day 11	
Breakfast	Omelette filled with diced tomatoes, onions, and feta cheese.
Snack	Handful of mixed nuts (almonds, walnuts, cashews).

Lunch	Grilled shrimp and avocado salad with mixed greens, cherry tomatoes, and balsamic vinaigrette.
Snack	Sliced cucumber with tzatziki sauce.
Dinner	Baked turkey meatballs with marinara sauce served over spaghetti squash.
Day 12	
Breakfast	Greek yogurt parfait with layers of mixed berries and granola.
Snack	Hard-boiled eggs.
Lunch	Chicken and vegetable stir-fry with snap peas, carrots, and broccoli served over brown rice.
Snack	Sliced bell peppers with guacamole.
Dinner	Grilled salmon fillets with roasted asparagus and quinoa.
Day 13	
Breakfast	Smoothie bowl topped with sliced kiwi, shredded coconut, and chia seeds.
Snack	Cottage cheese with pineapple chunks.

Lunch	Quinoa salad with black beans, corn, avocado, and cilantro. Dress with lime juice and olive oil.
Snack	Cherry tomatoes with mozzarella cheese.
Dinner	Baked chicken thighs with roasted Brussels sprouts and sweet potato wedges.

Day 14

Breakfast	Avocado toast on whole grain bread topped with sliced tomatoes and a sprinkle of sea salt.
Snack	Trail mix (dried fruit and nuts).
Lunch	Turkey and vegetable wraps with lettuce, cucumber, and hummus.
Snack	Sliced pear with cheese.
Dinner	Grilled lamb chops with roasted vegetables (carrots, parsnips, and turnips) and a side of quinoa pilaf.

Conclusion

In conclusion, understanding the unique dietary recommendations and metabolic tendencies associated with blood type O can empower individuals to make informed choices about their nutrition and overall health. By embracing a diet rich in high-quality proteins, beneficial fruits and vegetables, and healthy fats while avoiding lectin-rich foods and harmful ingredients, blood type O individuals can optimize their health and well-being.

Additionally, incorporating meal planning, preparation, and supplementation strategies tailored to individual needs and preferences can further support the success of a blood type O lifestyle. Whether it's designing balanced meal plans, batch cooking nutritious meals, or considering key supplements to address potential nutrient gaps, taking a proactive approach to nutrition can lead to long-term health benefits.

Furthermore, recognizing the importance of lifestyle factors such as stress management, regular physical activity, and adequate sleep can complement dietary efforts and contribute to overall wellness. By adopting a holistic approach to health that considers the interconnectedness of diet, lifestyle, and supplementation, blood type O individuals can embark on a journey towards sustained vitality and well-being.

In essence, the blood type O diet and lifestyle offer a framework for personalized nutrition and wellness that empowers individuals to take control of their health and thrive according to their unique genetic blueprint. Through mindful choices, informed decisions, and ongoing support, blood type O individuals can unlock their full potential and live life to the fullest.

Appendix

Blood Type O Food List

Reference Guide

	Beneficial Foods for Blood Type O:
1	High-Quality Proteins
	Lean cuts of beef, lamb, and venison.
	Poultry such as chicken and turkey.
	Fish such as salmon, cod, and mackerel.
	Shellfish including shrimp, lobster, and crab.
	Eggs, particularly from free-range or pasture-raised chickens.
2	Beneficial Fruits and Vegetables
	Dark leafy greens like kale, spinach, and Swiss chard.
	Cruciferous vegetables such as broccoli, Brussels sprouts, and cabbage.
	Berries including blueberries, blackberries, and raspberries.
	Apples, pears, and cherries.
	Pineapple, papaya, and figs.

3	Healthy Fats
	Olive oil, avocado oil, and flaxseed oil.
	Avocado.
	Nuts and seeds like almonds, walnuts, and flaxseeds.
	Coconut milk and coconut oil (in moderation).

Neutral Foods for Blood Type O:

1	Proteins
	Pork and bacon (in moderation).
	Lamb and goat cheese.
	Wild game like venison and pheasant.
	Most types of fish and seafood.
	Most types of beans and legumes.
2	Fruits and Vegetables
	Most fruits and vegetables not listed in the avoid category.
	Sweet potatoes and yams.
	Squash varieties like butternut and acorn squash.
	Peppers, onions, and garlic.
3	Healthy Fats

Ghee (clarified butter).

Sesame oil and sesame seeds.

Pumpkin seeds and sunflower seeds.

Butter (in moderation).

Foods to Avoid for Blood Type O

1 Proteins

Pork and pork products.

Certain types of seafood like octopus and caviar.

Processed meats like sausage and bacon.

Shellfish like clams and oysters.

2 Fruits and Vegetables

Oranges and orange juice.

Tomatoes and tomato-based products.

Nightshade vegetables such as potatoes, eggplant, and peppers.

Corn and corn products.

3 Grains and Legumes

Wheat and wheat products including bread and pasta.

Most types of grains like barley, rye, and oats.

	Legumes such as lentils, peanuts, and soybeans.
	Processed foods containing corn syrup and cornstarch.
Beverages	
Water is the best choice for hydration.	
Herbal teas, green tea, and occasional coffee (in moderation).	
Avoid sugary beverages, sodas, and fruit juices.	

Key Supplements to Consider

Supplements can be a valuable addition to the diet of blood type O individuals, providing targeted support for their unique metabolic tendencies and nutritional needs. While obtaining nutrients from whole foods is ideal, certain supplements may help fill potential gaps in the diet and support overall health and well-being. Here are some key supplements to consider for blood type O individuals:

1. Multivitamin and Mineral Supplements:

A high-quality multivitamin and mineral supplement can help ensure that blood type O individuals obtain essential nutrients that may be lacking in their diet. Look for a formulation specifically designed for blood type O, or choose a broad-spectrum supplement that includes vitamins and minerals such as vitamin D, vitamin B12, magnesium, zinc, and iron.

2. Omega-3 Fatty Acids:

Omega-3 fatty acids, particularly EPA (eicosapentaenoic acid) and DHA (docosahexaenoic acid), are essential fats that support cardiovascular health, brain function, and inflammation management. Blood type O individuals may benefit from supplementing with fish oil or algae-based omega-3 supplements to ensure an adequate intake of these beneficial fats.

3. Digestive Enzymes:

Blood type O individuals may have lower levels of stomach acid and reduced enzyme activity, which can affect digestion and nutrient absorption. Supplementing with digestive enzymes can help support efficient digestion and alleviate symptoms such as bloating, gas, and indigestion, particularly when consuming protein-rich meals or foods that may be challenging to digest.

4. Probiotics:

Maintaining a healthy balance of gut bacteria is essential for digestive health, immune function, and overall well-being. Blood type O individuals may benefit from supplementing with probiotics to support a healthy gut microbiome and alleviate digestive issues such as bloating, gas, and constipation. Look for a probiotic supplement that contains a variety of beneficial bacterial strains and has been specifically formulated for digestive health.

5. Adaptogenic Herbs:

Certain adaptogenic herbs such as ashwagandha, rhodiola, and ginseng may help support stress management, energy levels, and hormonal balance in blood type O individuals. These herbs have been traditionally used to promote resilience to stress and enhance overall vitality. Consider incorporating adaptogenic herbs into your supplement regimen to support your body's natural response to stress and promote overall well-being.

6. Vitamin D:

Many people, including blood type O individuals, may have insufficient levels of vitamin D due to limited sun exposure and dietary intake. Vitamin D plays a crucial role in bone health, immune function, and mood regulation. Supplementing with vitamin D, particularly during the winter months or if you have limited sun exposure, can help maintain optimal levels and support overall health.

7. Magnesium:

Magnesium is an essential mineral involved in hundreds of biochemical reactions in the body, including muscle function, nerve transmission, and energy production. Blood type O individuals may benefit from supplementing with magnesium to support muscle relaxation, stress management, and overall wellness. Choose a magnesium supplement that is well-absorbed and bioavailable, such as magnesium citrate or magnesium glycinate.

www.ingramcontent.com/pod-product-compliance
Lightning Source LLC
Chambersburg PA
CBHW071551260726
48653CB00007BA/2719